Smile BIG!

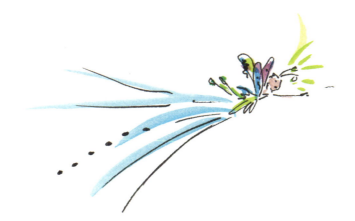

What Happened to the Tooth Fairy?

By Graham Gardner

Illustrated by Nancy LeBlanc

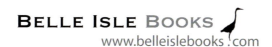

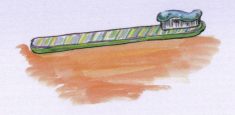

This special book belongs especially to

Copyright 2014 by Graham Gardner. No portion of this book may be reproduced or transmitted in any form whatsoever without prior written permission from the publisher, except in the case of brief quotations published in articles and reviews.

ISBN: 978-1-9399301-5-6

Library of Congress Control Number: 2013954284

Published by
BELLE ISLE BOOKS
www.belleislebooks.com

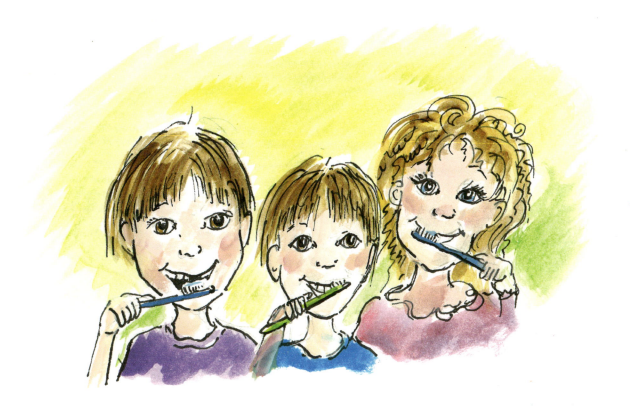

To Ava, Finn, and Oliver. Please brush your teeth.

Oliver sat straight up in bed. It was Saturday morning, and he remembered that just yesterday he had lost a tooth! Last night, he'd put the tooth in his special tooth fairy box and left it under his pillow. He couldn't wait to see what the tooth fairy had brought him!

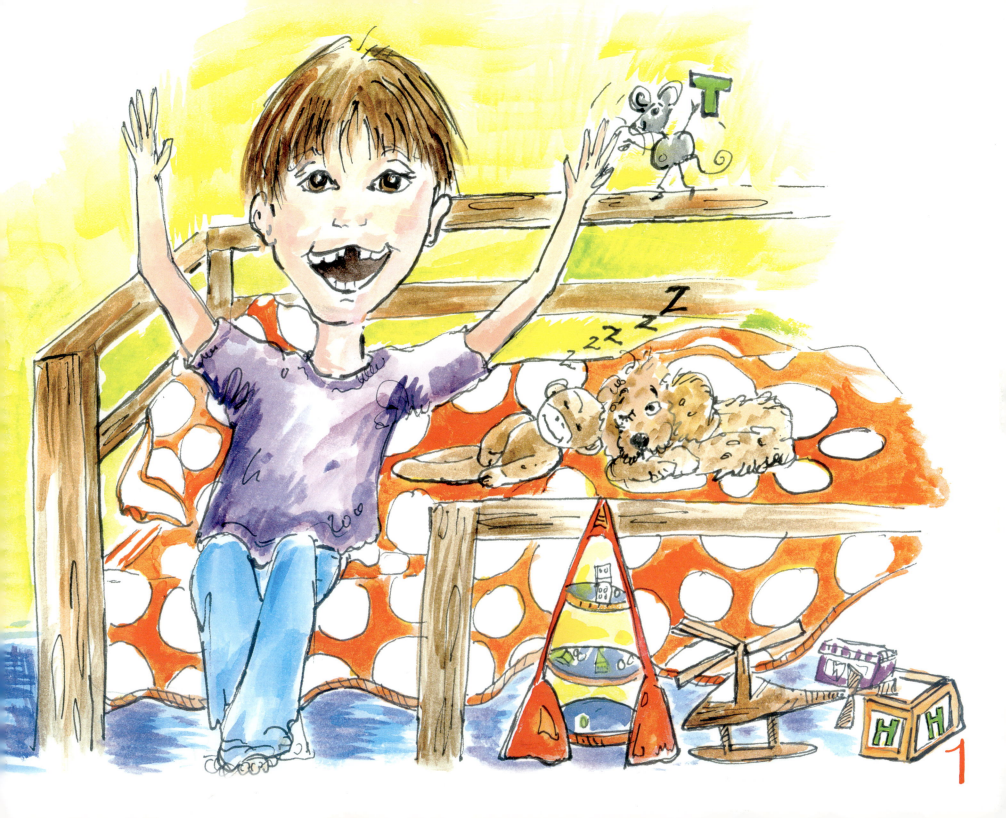

Oliver felt under his pillow for his tooth fairy box, but he couldn't find it.

He threw his pillow on the floor and dove under his sheets. Still he found nothing.

Then he looked under his bed, and there it was! Whew! His tooth fairy box was on the floor beside his wooden helicopter.

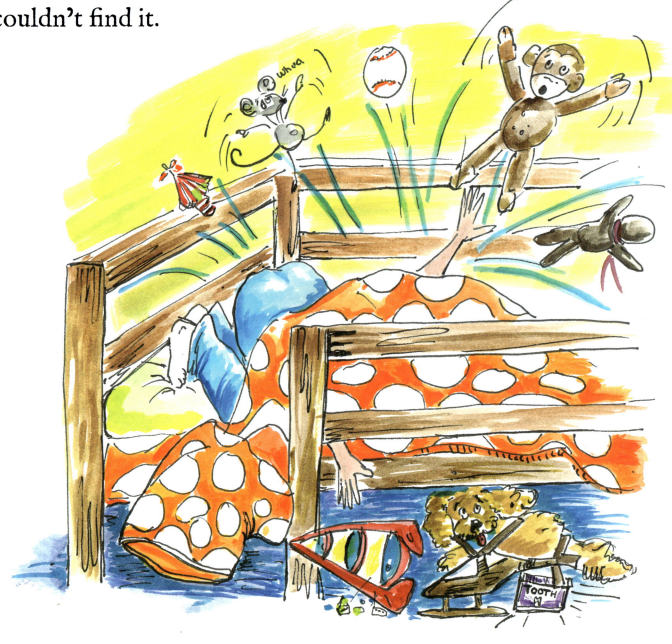

Oliver grabbed it and opened it. He couldn't believe his eyes!
There, in his little tooth fairy box, nestled in tissue, was . . . his tooth!

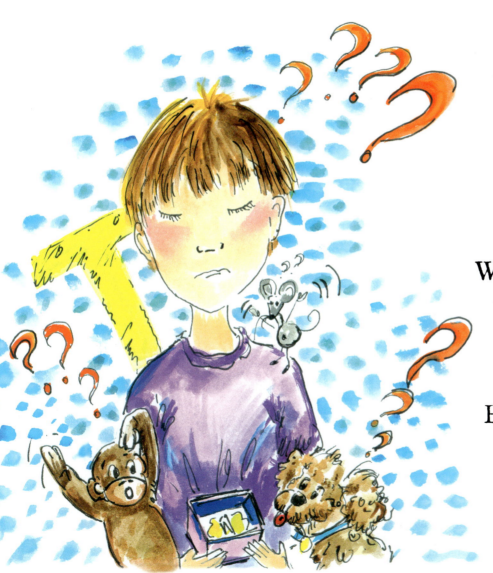

Not a coin like he had expected, not a crisp dollar bill, but his big front tooth!

What had happened?
Why hadn't the tooth fairy come?
Oliver needed to know.

Had he done something wrong?
Was the tooth fairy hurt?

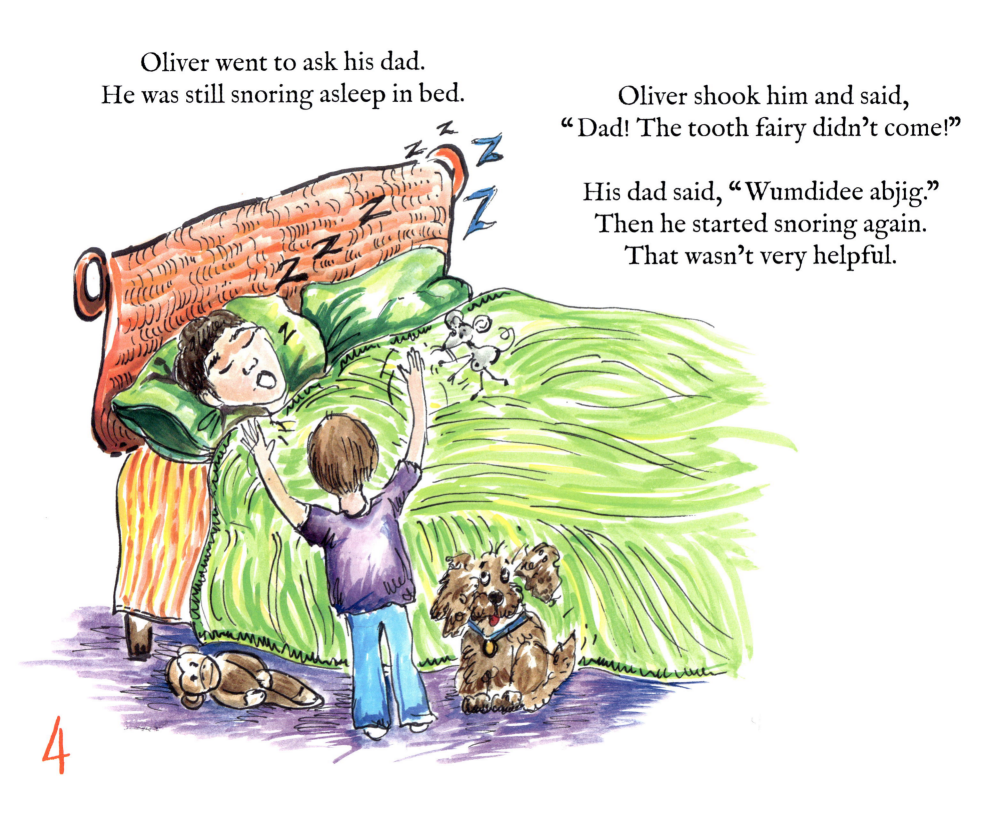

Oliver went to ask his dad.
He was still snoring asleep in bed.

Oliver shook him and said,
"Dad! The tooth fairy didn't come!"

His dad said, "Wumdidee abjig."
Then he started snoring again.
That wasn't very helpful.

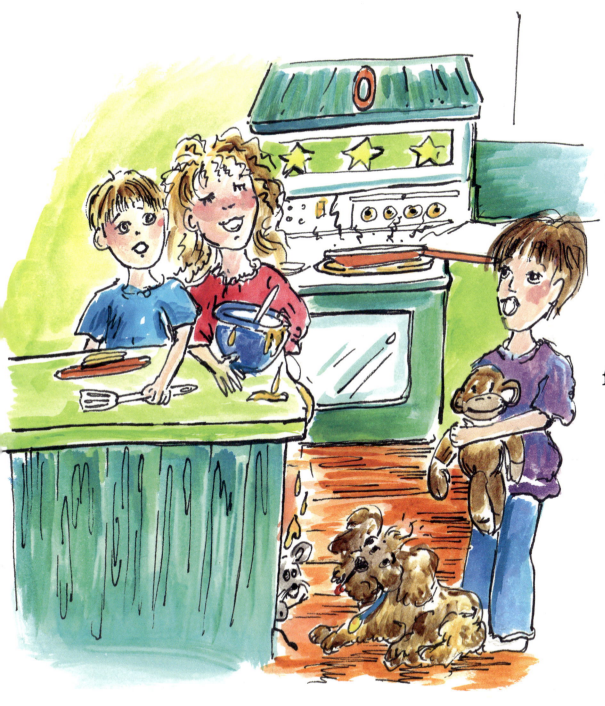

Oliver went to ask his sister and brother, who were making breakfast for their dad.

His sister said, "That happened to me once, but she came the next night."

That was good to hear, but it didn't explain why the tooth fairy hadn't come the first night.

"But why didn't she come right away?" Oliver asked.

His sister and brother looked curiously at Oliver. "We don't know," they replied together.

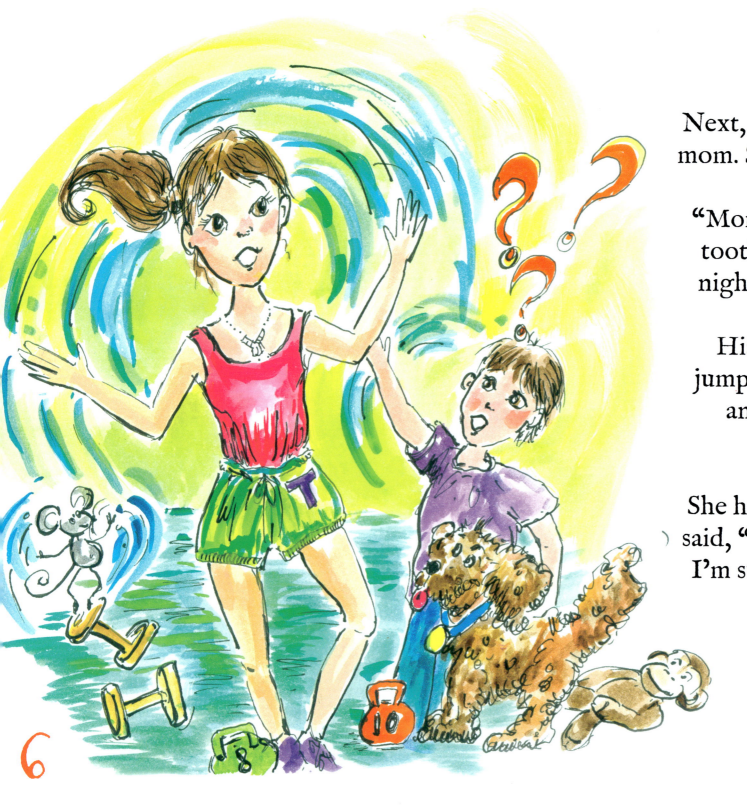

Next, Oliver went to his mom. She was exercising.

"Mom, why didn't the tooth fairy come last night?" Oliver asked.

His mom stopped jumping up and down and looked very surprised.

She hugged Oliver and said, "I don't know, but I'm sure she will come tonight."

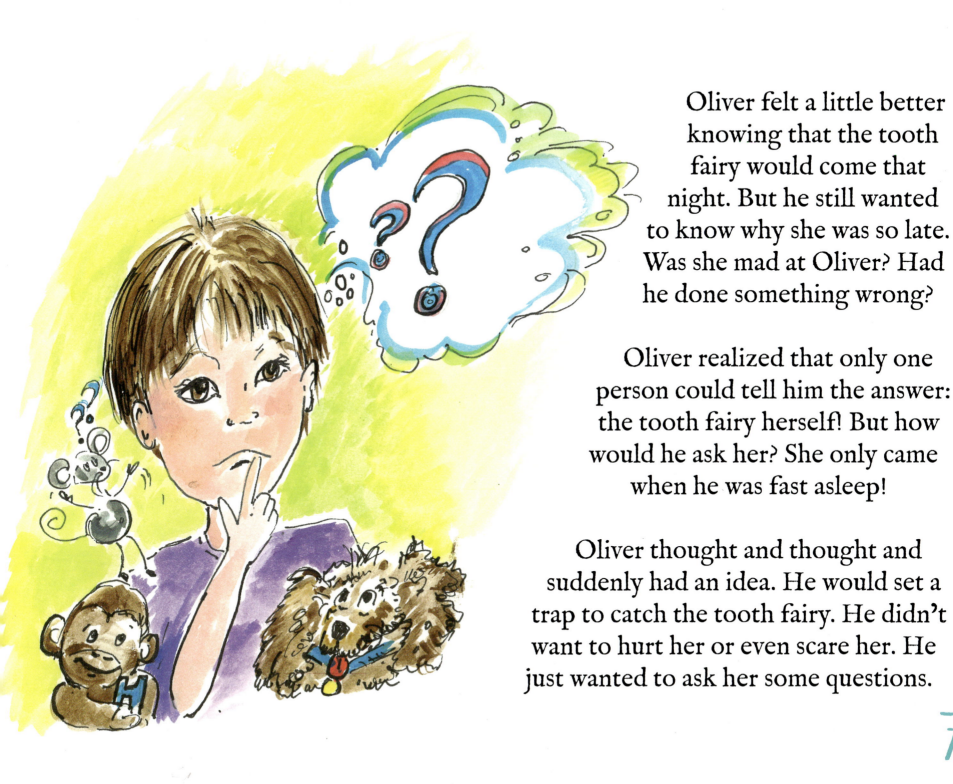

Oliver felt a little better knowing that the tooth fairy would come that night. But he still wanted to know why she was so late. Was she mad at Oliver? Had he done something wrong?

Oliver realized that only one person could tell him the answer: the tooth fairy herself! But how would he ask her? She only came when he was fast asleep!

Oliver thought and thought and suddenly had an idea. He would set a trap to catch the tooth fairy. He didn't want to hurt her or even scare her. He just wanted to ask her some questions.

So he got a shoebox and attached a plastic cup to it with some tape. Then he added a spring and some straws and a wooden spoon.

He worked all day on his project. He put some cereal in the trap because he thought the tooth fairy might like that.

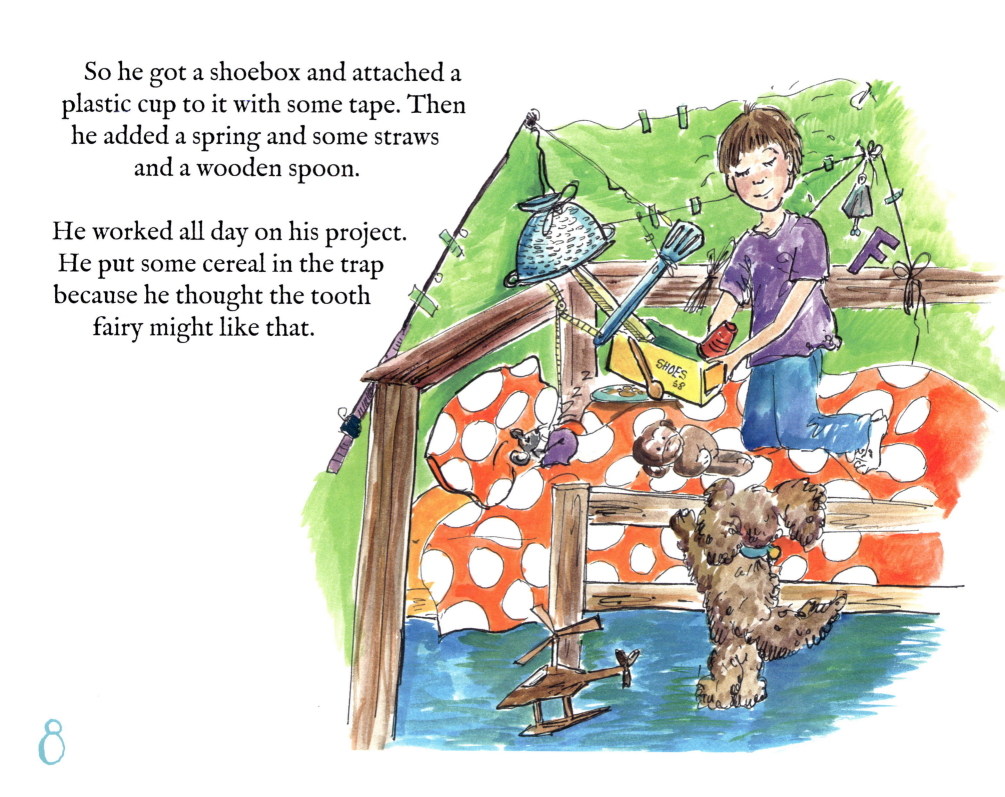

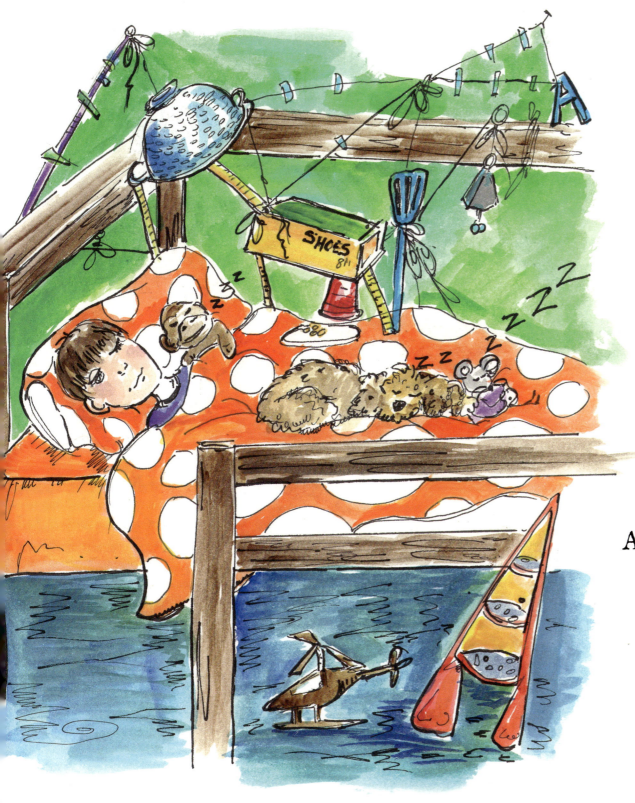

When Oliver went to bed, he was so excited that he stayed awake for a long time.

A few minutes before midnight, he finally ...
fell ...
asleep ...

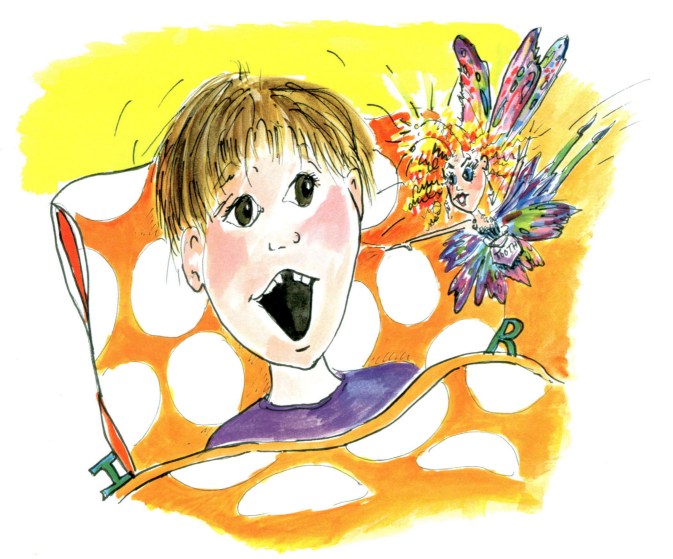

Suddenly, Oliver felt a tug on his ear. He opened one eye to see what it was. Standing on his pillow in front of his nose was a tiny, beautiful woman no bigger than his hand. She had two antennae sprouting from her head, and wings like a dragonfly's. She also had a very stern look on her face.
"Hey, Oliver!" she said. "Don't you know that you can't catch the tooth fairy?"

Oliver was so surprised, it took him a moment to answer.
"I just wanted to know why you didn't come last night.
I was worried," he said.

The tooth fairy giggled. "You are sweet to worry about me,
Oliver. I was just fine. You must understand that I'm a very
small fairy and it's a very big world, with lots of children
losing teeth every day. I try my best to be on time, but there
are so many reasons I can't make it to every house when
I'm supposed to."

Oliver hadn't thought about all the other children losing
teeth in the world. She certainly was a small fairy.

Oliver was curious. "What are some of the reasons?" he asked.

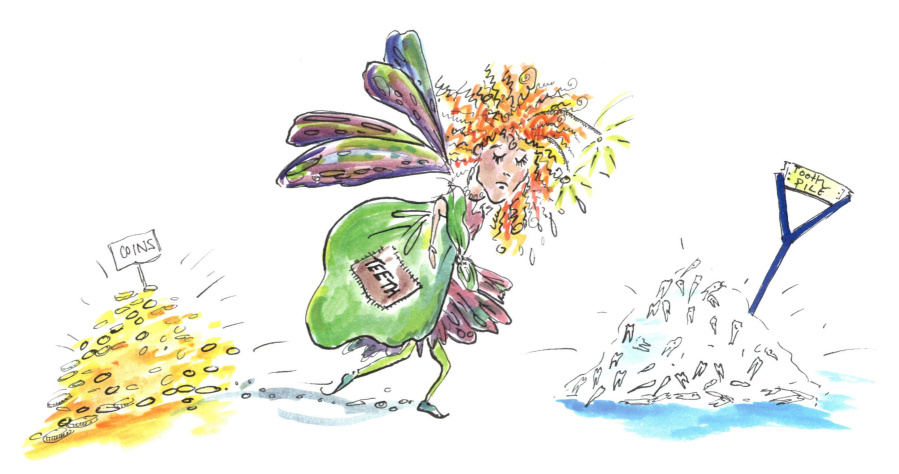

"The most common reason is that sometimes too many children lose a tooth on the same night. I can only carry so many teeth and coins at a time, and I can only go to so many houses in one night."

Oliver nodded. That made a lot of sense.
The tooth fairy began walking back and forth on Oliver's pillow, explaining the reasons why she was sometimes not able to get children's teeth.

"If a child loses a tooth too late in the day, I might not have time to add it to my pick-up list," she explained. "And when children are up too late, sometimes I have to move on to the next child, because I can't just wait around all night for one child when others are waiting."

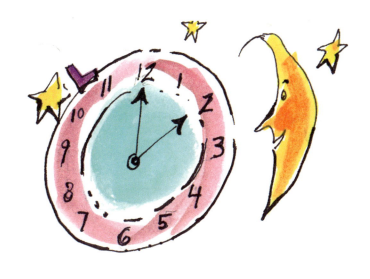

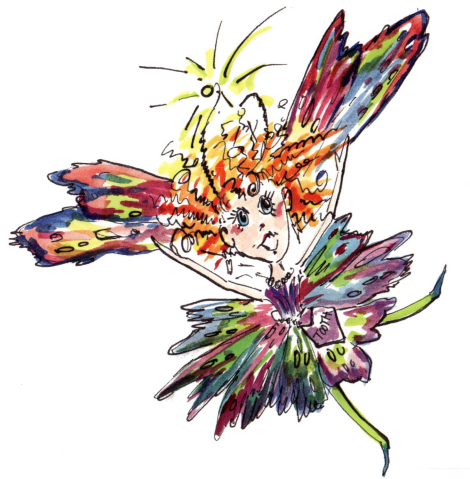

Oliver nodded again. That made sense, too. But it was late, and he was getting sleepy, so he put his head back on his pillow to listen some more.

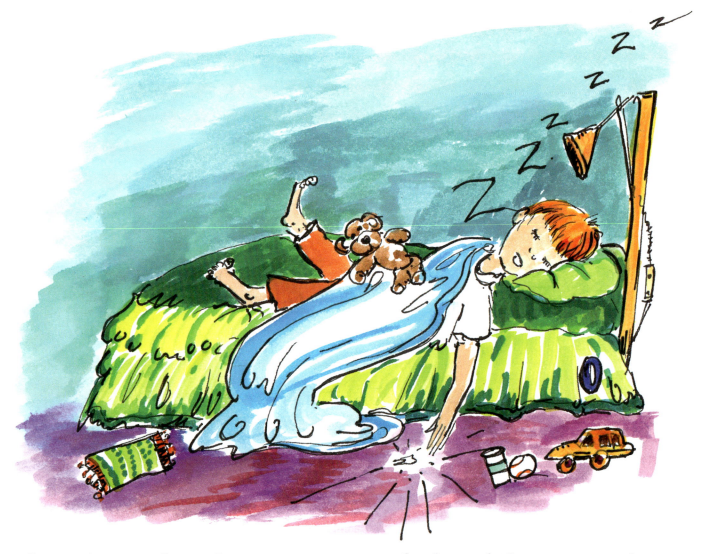

"Did you know that if you move around a lot while you are sleeping, you can push your tooth off of your bed?" the tooth fairy said. "You should have your mom or dad check to see that the tooth is still in place after you go to sleep."

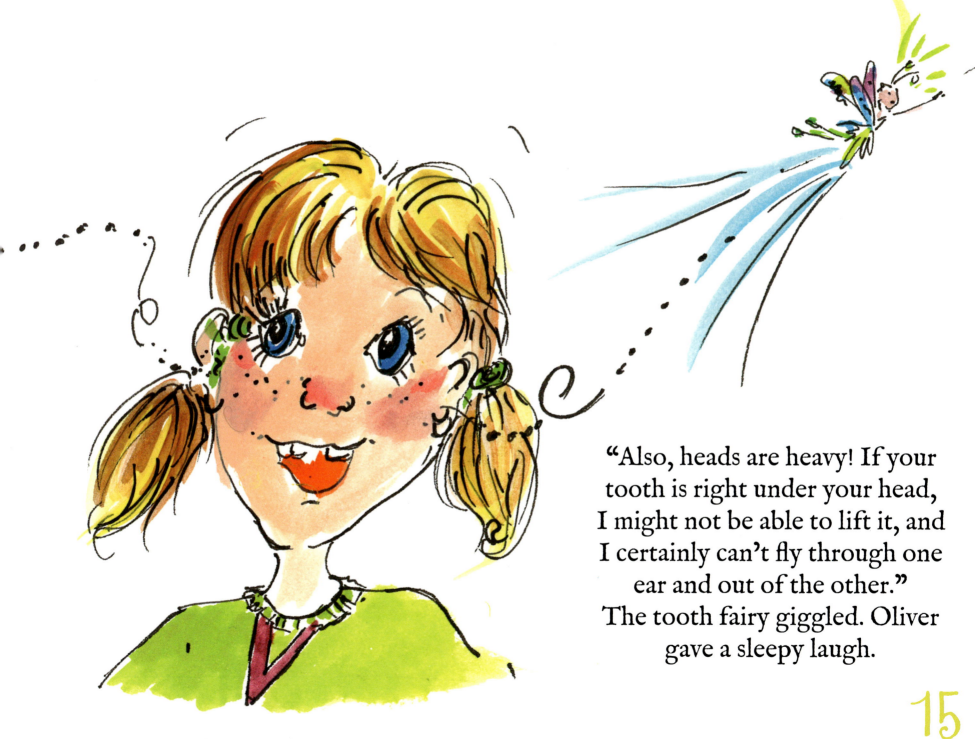

"Also, heads are heavy! If your tooth is right under your head, I might not be able to lift it, and I certainly can't fly through one ear and out of the other."
The tooth fairy giggled. Oliver gave a sleepy laugh.

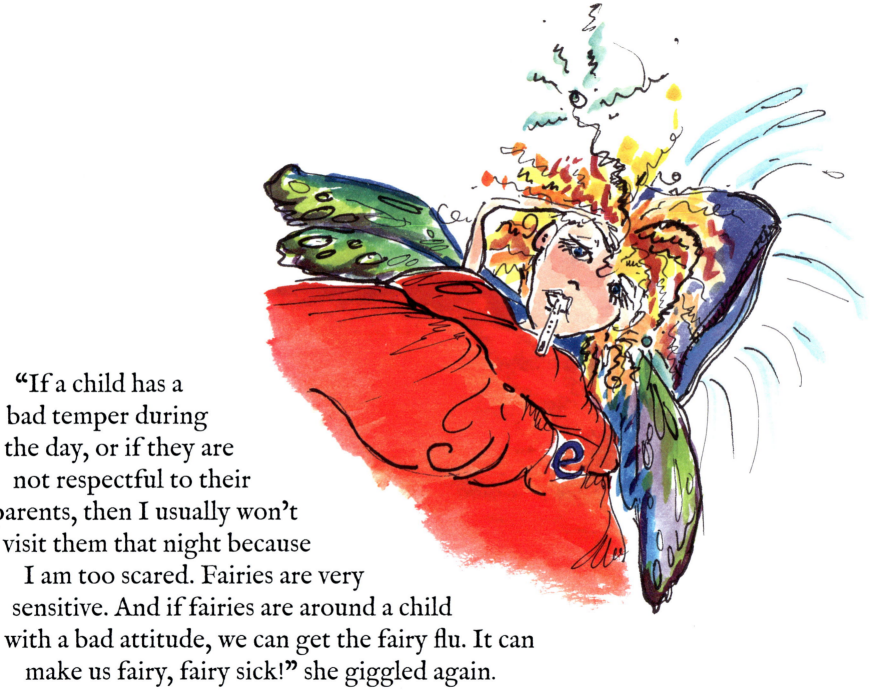

"If a child has a bad temper during the day, or if they are not respectful to their parents, then I usually won't visit them that night because I am too scared. Fairies are very sensitive. And if fairies are around a child with a bad attitude, we can get the fairy flu. It can make us fairy, fairy sick!" she giggled again.

"If someone has a messy room, sometimes I have to give the money to their parents to pay them for cleaning up the room."

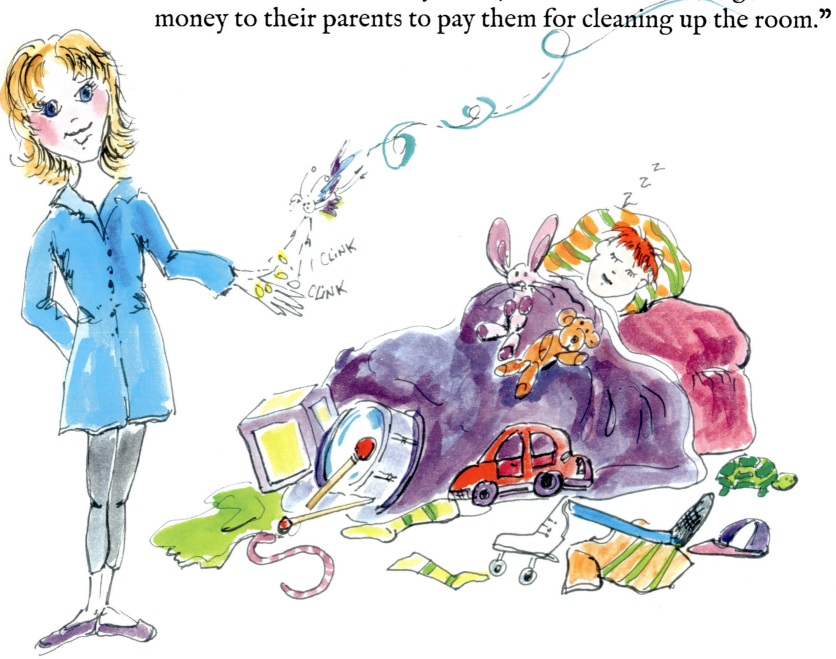

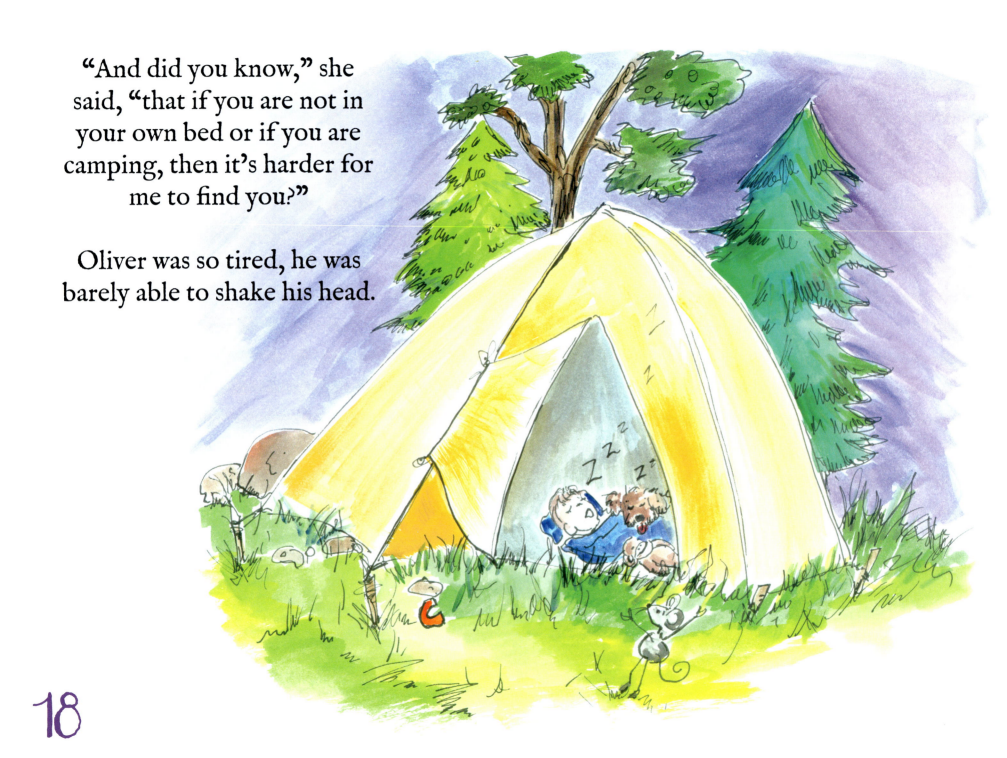

"And did you know," she said, "that if you are not in your own bed or if you are camping, then it's harder for me to find you?"

Oliver was so tired, he was barely able to shake his head.

"Sometimes, things happen to make me late," the tooth fairy continued.
"One time I got caught in the strings of a fairy mobile hanging over a child's bed. I was stuck there for two days until another fairy freed me. I blended in with the wooden fairies on the mobile, so nobody noticed me."

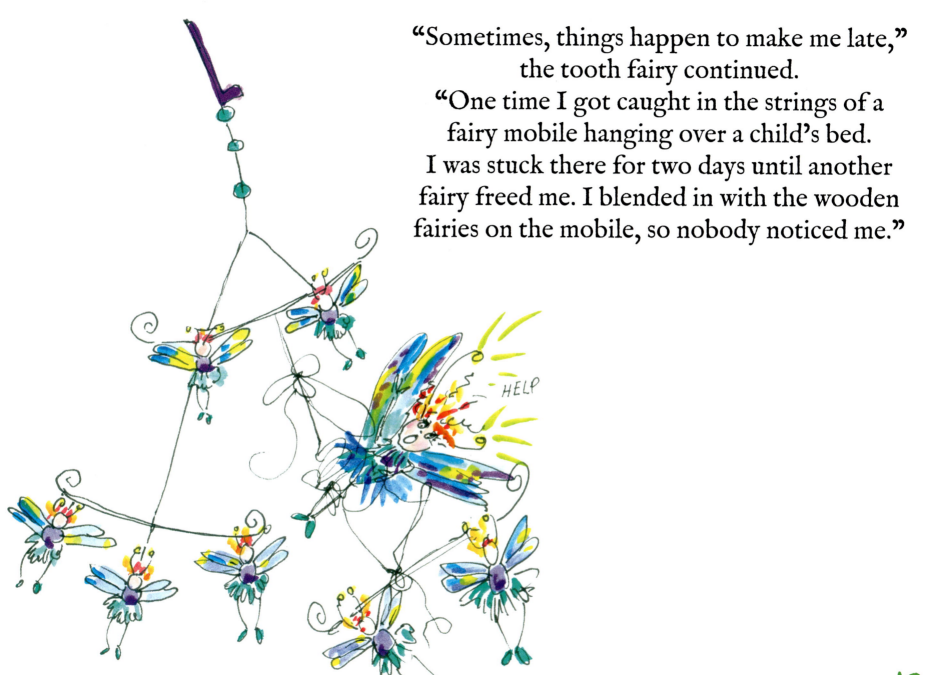

"Most people don't know this," she whispered in Oliver's ear, "but fairies shed wings just like children lose teeth, one at a time. A new one grows back quickly, but until it does, I can only fly in circles, which slows me down. Once the new wing is grown, I can fly faster than ever, though, which helps me catch up."

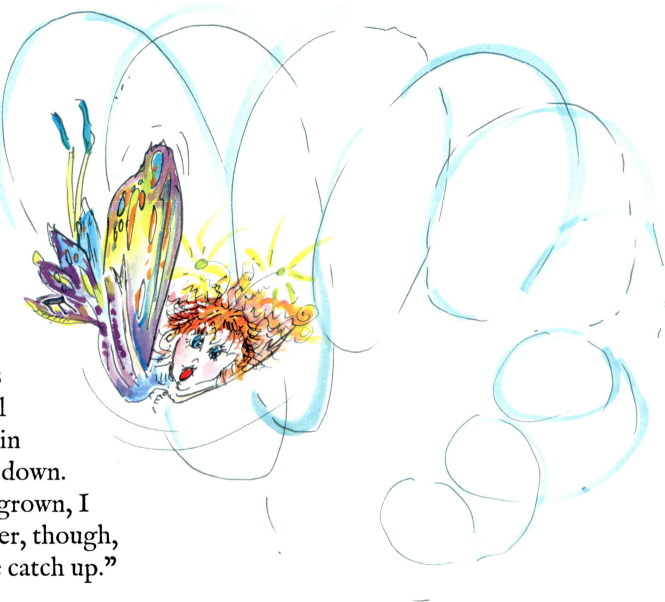

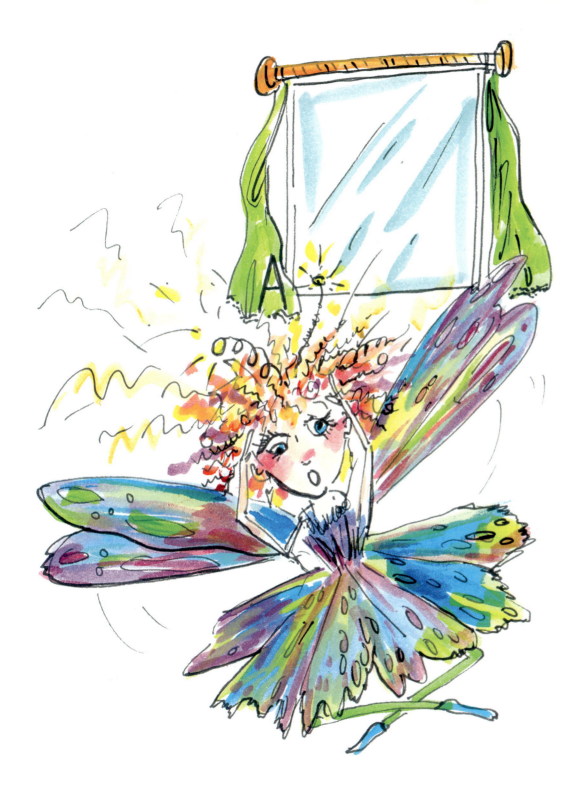

"One of the worst problems that caused me to be late is when I thought a window was open but it wasn't. I ran straight into it and broke my antennae. I was lost for days because I was so dizzy. Some children who had not even lost a tooth got money!"

Oliver's eyes were closed now, but he smiled drowsily at that.

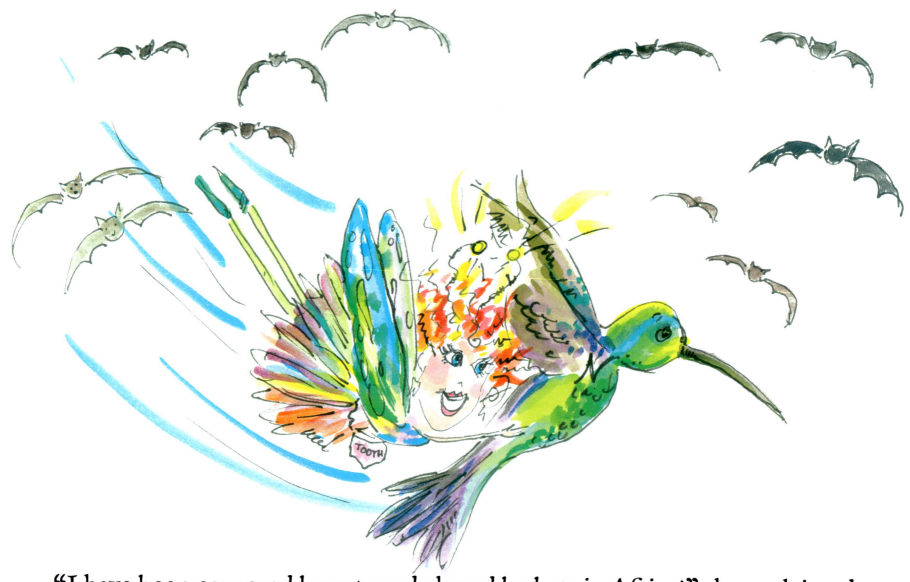

"I have been cornered by cats and chased by bats in Africa!" she exclaimed. "I hit a tree once flying away from bats and broke a wing. Luckily a hummingbird gave me a ride for several days as it healed." She added with a whisper, "Hummingbirds are nice, but they are very slow compared to fairies."

"In your case, however," she said with a smile, "I didn't come last night because my friends threw a surprise party for me. You see, yesterday was my birthday!"

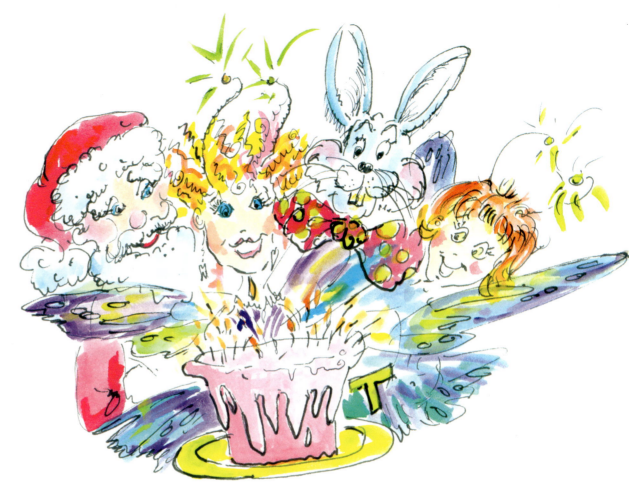

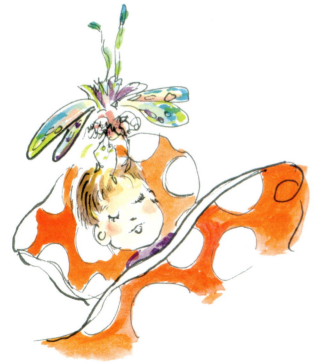

She looked at Oliver, expecting him to say "Happy Birthday," and suddenly realized that he had fallen asleep.
"Good night, sweet child," she said.

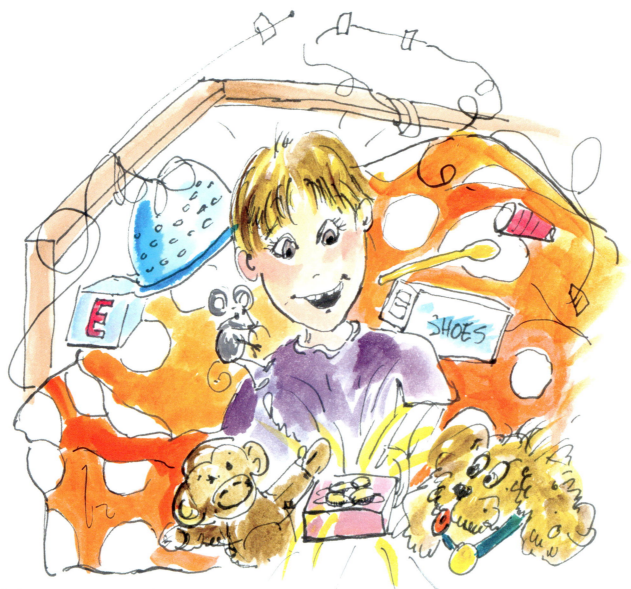

When Oliver awoke the next morning, he remembered his visit from the tooth fairy. He looked at his trap. It had fallen apart. He quickly opened his tooth fairy box. Inside the box there were four shiny quarters.

Oliver was so excited that he went to tell his brother and sister. But first he wrote the tooth fairy a nice thank you note.

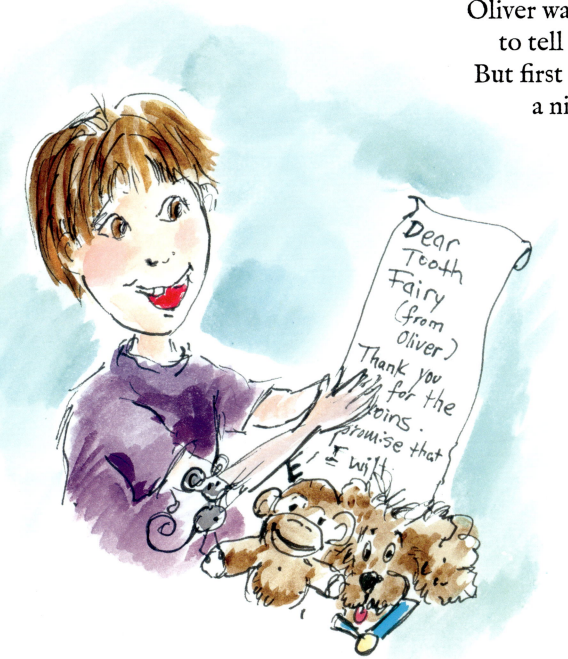

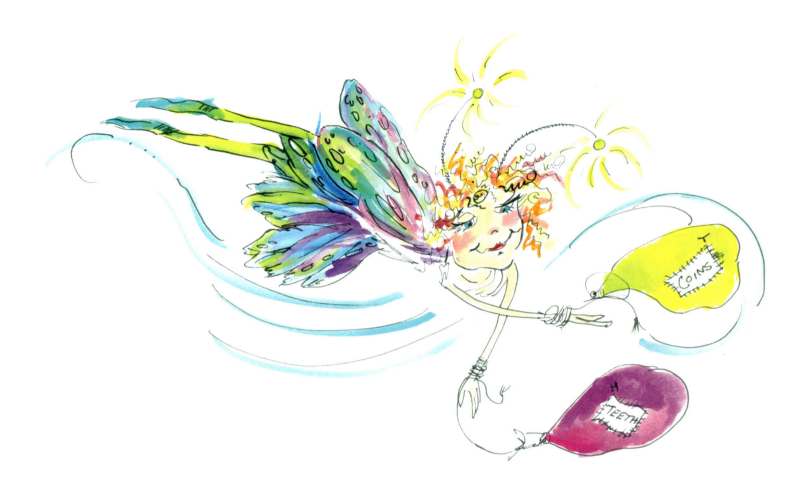

Oliver lost many more teeth after that, and sometimes the tooth fairy came right away, and sometimes she was late. But Oliver never worried. He knew she was very busy. And, to tell the truth, he suspected she was a little bit scatterbrained, too.

THE END!
Sleep well and have wonderful dreams.

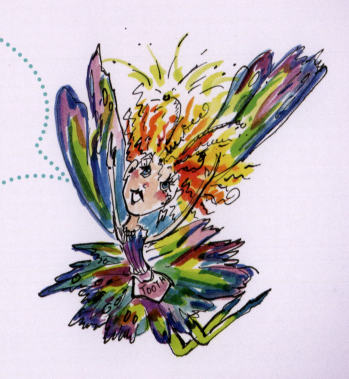

Go back and find the hidden letters on each page to spell out a secret message.

Secret Message:

¡hteeT naelC sevoL yriaF htooT ehT

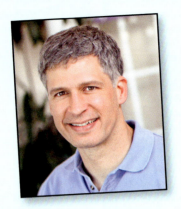

Graham Gardner

Graham was born in West Berlin on an American army base, grew up in a beautiful little town called Martinsville, Virginia, and now lives in Richmond, Virginia with his family in a very strange house on the river. He received his degree in dentistry at Virginia Commonwealth University, and became an orthodontist at New York University, so he gets to help people with their smiles every day. Graham loves spending time with his family, kite boarding and whitewater kayaking but most of all, he loves life! Graham is also published in orthodontic scientific publications, where he writes about the importance of having a great smile. He hopes this book will make you smile, too!

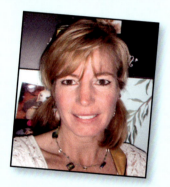

Nancy Cecere-LeBlanc

Nancy LeBlanc was born and grew up in New Jersey and studied art therapy and art education. While volunteering, working odd jobs and raising her children, she has continued to work on her art in a variety of ways, including painting walls and furniture, and making jewelry. Two things have always remained constant in Nancy's life, and that is her love of animals and her love of art. For many years, she has volunteered with a local canine rescue organization, which continues to inspire her work. She now paints pet portraits and works on her own studies of farm animals and other things that spark her fancy. She currently lives in Henrico, Virginia with her husband, three children and various animals.

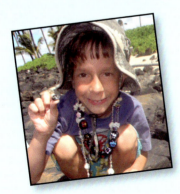

Oliver Gardner

Oliver is a big ball of positive creative energy! If there was a blackout in New York City, you could plug him in and light Times Square. He rocks the harmonica and is probably the funniest person you'll ever meet. Oliver is a champion reader and a computer guru. He overcame all odds at birth, which earned him the middle name of Atlas. He inspires his father, who is very very proud of him.